my
health
theory

jonathan **mclaughlin**
órla **mclaughlin**

Copyright

Visit the authors' website at www.my**health**theory.com

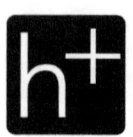

improve
your
health

About the authors

Jonathan and Órla McLaughlin are a brother-and-sister team who have spent a considerable amount of time over the past three years working on my **health** theory.

Jonathan is a published mathematician while Órla is a practicing nutritionist and it is this combination of concise structured thinking and in-depth practical knowledge which has resulted in my **health** theory.

About the book

We now set out some basic points about the style of *my **health** theory*.

- A minimalistic approach has been taken to both the style and the language used in *my **health** theory*.

- The basic facts on each topic are laid out in the understanding that you will fill in the details.

- There is no prescriptive aspect to *my **health** theory*, we do not promote any *best* type of healthy lifestyle.

- You can think of *my **health** theory* as a guide book as you work your way towards a healthier lifestyle.

- There is plenty of white space in *my **health** theory* and you are encouraged to scribble notes in these spaces as you work your way through the book.

Introduction

Introduction

The main aim of *my **health** theory* can be described by this three word slogan:

improve **your** health

This book sets out to improve your health by guiding you towards living a healthier lifestyle.

A variety of topics are presented so that you can decide the exact combination of these topics which are most relevant to your health.

There are lots and lots of healthy lifestyles and no single healthy lifestyle is perfect. However, there may well be a perfect healthy lifestyle **for you.**

This is a key point in *my **health** theory,* you must personalise any healthy lifestyle to suit your needs.

Your current state of health is not important as there is always room for improvement.

The two simple requirements before starting *my **health** theory* are your desire and your commitment to improve your health.

So, let's go!

A starting analogy

Consider building your perfect home:

1. First of all, you would look at other homes to get ideas and inspiration.
2. Then you would draw up a set of blueprints.
3. After that you would then build your home.
4. Finally, you would live happily ever after in your perfect home!

Each of the four respective steps can be described by a single word as follows:

1. Research
2. Plan
3. Implement
4. Maintain

A starting analogy

Now consider the previous four steps when building your perfect healthy lifestyle.

It is vital that all four steps are considered.

During Step 1 you will find inspiration and ideas for your perfect healthy lifestyle.

In Step 2 you will plan out your perfect healthy lifestyle, paying particular attention to how you will be able to maintain this lifestyle.

In Step 3 you will make all the changes to your lifestyle which you set out in the plan that you drew in Step 2.

Finally, you will then be able to start Step 4, living happily and healthily ever after!

Structure

This book contains four parts:

1. **Principles**
   This part of the book sets out the fundamental ideas which underpin the remainder of the book.

2. **Tools**
   This part contains the basic methods that you need to effectively analyse the information needed to construct your health theory.

3. **Framework**
   This part acts as a guide or framework for your research and outlines the main factors which you might consider when designing your health theory.

4. **My health theory**
   You will construct your own personal health theory with all of the information you have gathered during your research. *This is the most important part of the book*!

Principles

Basic principles

A *principle* is a fundamental truth which serves as a foundation for a system or theory.

A collection of principles on which the practice of an activity is built is called a *theory* or a *philosophy*.

This book is built on the following basic principles:
- Clarity
- Objectivity
- Commitment
- Practicality

We will now examine each of these principles in turn.

Before we can design a perfect healthy lifestyle we must first ask the question:

What is health?

To answer this question we will use the definition that the World Health Organisation (WHO) has used since 1948:

Health is a state of complete physical, mental and social well-being and not merely the absence of disease or infirmity.

Note the **three** distinct aspects of this definition:

1. Physical well-being
2. Mental well-being
3. Social well-being

Therefore, it is clear that any worthwhile health theory will consist of much more than simply eating a few more vegetables and perhaps some running.

Objectivity

To ensure a high quality health theory it is vital to use only high quality factual information.

Information is **objective** if it is unbiased and based only on facts.

Information is **subjective** if it is based on opinion or on personal feelings, tastes or other preconceptions.

You should aim to make your health theory as objective as possible.

Of course, in reality, information is rarely either objective or subjective but rather somewhere between the two.

Deciding the level of objectivity or subjectivity in a particular statement is a key skill that will be required when designing your health theory and perfect healthy lifestyle.

Objectivity, opinion & choice

It will be necessary to use your opinion as you find and analyse information.

Therefore, it is unavoidable that your health theory will contain some level of subjectivity.

This means that your opinion will play an important role in your health theory.

As a result, it is vital that your opinion is:
- clear
- well-informed
- as objective as possible

You will make a multitude of choices as you attempt to find a workable and achievable balance in every aspect of your health theory.

These choices will be based on your opinion, as well as on your research.

It is therefore vital to reiterate the point that your opinion is well-informed, clear and balanced so that each choice that you make is as objective as possible.

Objectivity & preconceptions

Your opinions are influenced by your preconceptions i.e. the views which you currently consider to be true.

Examining your relevant preconceptions to determine if they are in fact true will be vital.

Always ask:

Why is this true?

Remember that any view, if it is correct, will stand up to a detailed examination.

Science never fears scrutiny!

Obstacles to objectivity

Common obstacles to an unbiased opinion include:

1. **Your ego**
   You may disregard evidence against your current view in case this view is shown to be wrong, which may then dent your ego.

2. **Your allegiances**
   Your current allegiance to some school-of-thought may cause you to disregard evidence which contradicts this school-of-thought.

3. **Ambiguity**
   It is vital to know the exact meaning of every word in the question you are attempting to answer. A vague understanding is not enough. Science does not allow ambiguity.

Commitment & excuses

Your healthy lifestyle will require commitment.

The greater your commitment to designing and implementing your health theory the higher the likelihood that you will achieve beneficial results after reading this book.

It is important to recognise and then avoid excuses.

Excuses are the biggest threat to your commitment.

Make changes, not excuses!

Four assumptions

Consider the following four simple assumptions when designing your health theory:

1. **No single best health theory exists**
   - Two people can have wildly different, but equally good health theories.
   - Remember, what is perfect for you may not suit someone else, and vice versa.

2. **No simplistic or short health theory exists**
   - Your health is not just determined by one or two factors, it is in fact influenced by a myriad of different factors.
   - As a result, any worthwhile health theory must involve the careful consideration of many factors.

3. **No effortless health theory exists**
   - Rarely is the easiest option the best option.
   - Effort will be required!

4. **No quick health theory exists**
   - The main goal of this book is for you to design your perfect healthy lifestyle which you can implement in your daily life, indefinitely.
   - There should be no elements of "fad-diets" or "quick-fixes" in any useful health theory.
   - Sustainability is the keyword here.

Practicality

A key point to note is that any health theory, no matter how well researched, designed and constructed, is of little or no value if it is not practical.

We now examine the following issues which may affect the practicality of your health theory:
- Pleasure
- Extremes
- Balance
- Flexibility
- Time & money

Failing to consider these issues may significantly reduce both the practicality and the sustainability, and hence the overall value, of your health theory.

Practicality
Pleasure

For almost everyone, pleasure is one of, if not *the*, main motivating factor in many situations.

Overlooking pleasure in your health theory will render your theory practically worthless.

Consider the following aspects of pleasure:

1. **Taste**
   Some might say the nicer the taste the less healthy the option and so some sort of compromise may be necessary here.

2. **Physical effort and relaxation**
   Frequently the most desirable option requires less effort than alternative healthier choices. Again, a balance will need to be struck.

3. **Enjoyment**
   If we enjoy an activity then generally we continue doing it. If such an activity is deemed unhealthy then it may be advisable to reduce the time spent on this activity with a view to perhaps eventually stopping the activity altogether.

Practicality
Extremes

A common factor in many popular diet books or fitness plans is some sort of extreme.

These books and plans are commonly accompanied by phrases such as "only do this" or "never do that".

It is worth noting however, that extremes can be considered unnatural in some sense.

For example, few people live in the Arctic or in the Sahara.

The most relevant aspect of extremes is that they are difficult to maintain in the long term.

As a result, it may not be a good idea to incorporate extreme options into your health theory but instead choose less drastic alternatives which are more sustainable.

Practicality
Balance

Unlike extremes, balance and equilibrium are more natural phenomena.

In fact, equilibrium is a key concept in:
- Physics
- Biology
- Chemistry
- Economics

It is therefore highly likely that the sustainability of your health theory will be greatly enhanced by incorporating the concept of balance.

Practicality
Flexibility

Life rarely sticks to a timetable.

As a result, you must be able to adapt to your constantly changing circumstances, and so must your health theory.

Of course any useful health theory must be practical and sustainable but just as importantly, your health theory must also have the ability to adapt to changes in your day-to-day life.

Therefore, your health theory will require some degree of in-built flexibility.

Practicality
Time & money

There are two great scarcities in life:

1. **Time**

2. **Money**

When designing your sustainable health theory it is imperative that due consideration is given to both these factors.

A useful health theory cannot place unrealistic demands on your time.

Equally true is the observation that a useful health theory must be affordable.

Like the blueprints for your perfect home mentioned at the start of the book, if the house will take 10 years and $10 million to build, then those blueprints are unlikely to be very useful to you.

Tools

Tools

To build your perfect home a wide range of machinery, tools and skills are needed.

The design, construction and implementation of your health theory will be no different.

Some of the most useful tools which you will need are:
- Common sense
- Finding useful information
- Decision making
- Motivation
- Professional help

We will now examine each of these tools in turn.

Common sense

It will be of the utmost importance that you use logical, step-by-step reasoning when you are designing and constructing your health theory i.e. you must use your common sense.

Logical reasoning will be used to combine various facts in a logical way with the goal of reaching a sensible conclusion. This conclusion must follow directly from these combined facts.

Logical reasoning will also be used to turn evidence or observations into a plausible theory which can then be tested.

To this end, a later subsection of the book is dedicated to conducting your own trials.

Finding information

Today, finding information is not a problem.

Vast quantities of information can be obtained from:
- the internet
- printed media
- lectures and talks
- conversations

However, finding high quality, useful information can be a problem.

As a result, the issue of determining the quality of information is addressed in the coming pages.

When searching the internet it may be useful to "bookmark" webpages which you find useful so that you can quickly and easily revisit them in the future.

As was mentioned at the beginning of the book, there is lots of white space in this book and you are encouraged to fill this space with your thoughts, views and other interesting information that you have found.

Analysing information

Having found information, it must then be analysed to determine its usefulness.

Useful information must be both:
- relevant
- trustworthy

Determining the relevance of information should be fairly straightforward as long as you have a clear question which you wish to answer.

However, determining the trustworthiness of a piece of information can be trickier.

Consequently, much of the remainder of this section is dedicated to analysing the trustworthiness of information.

Types of information

When considering any piece of information you should try to classify it into one of the following 4 categories:

1. A **fact** is a piece of information supported by a clear logical explanation as to why it is true. A fact is the most trustworthy piece of information.

2. A **result** is a piece of information supported by a large volume of experimental and observational evidence. Sometimes there may be no generally accepted explanation as to why this piece of information is thought to be true. A result is quite a trustworthy piece of information.

3. A **finding** is a piece of information found in a single or small number of experiments or observations and there is no explanation as to why this piece of information may be true. A finding should always be treated with a degree of doubt.

4. An **opinion** is a piece of information which is a personal view and may or may not be supported by facts, results and/or findings. Treat all opinions with at least some degree of scepticism.

When constructing your health theory you should aim to include more facts than results, more results than findings and more findings than opinions.

Sources of information

It is important to remember that the source of any piece of information can greatly affect the trustworthiness of the information.

When analysing a piece of information you should ask the following questions:

- Is the information written by the original researcher or is it relayed or summarised by someone else?

- Do you sense that the author is trying to convince you of something? Note that proper scientific writing should be objective rather than persuasive.

- Who funded the research or paid the author? Might there be any potential conflict of interest?

- How much, if any, of the information is based on the author's opinion?

Scientific studies

When reading the conclusions of scientific studies the basis of these conclusion should be clearly stated.

Establish if the conclusion of the study is based on:
- survey/questionnaire data
- experimental data
- logical explanation
- or some combination of the above three

When a pattern occurs in data related to two different events, then a statistical relationship is said to exist between the two events.

A very important note must now be made about statistical relationships.
- When the reason for the statistical relationship between the events is logically **explained** then there is a **causal** relationship between the events.
- If the statistical relationship is simply **observed**, but not explained, then there is merely a **correlation** between the events.

Note that finding a correlation does **not** guarantee that there is a causal relationship.

Conclusions based on correlations are **much weaker** than conclusions based on the logical explanation of a causal relationship.

Making comparisons

Making comparisons will be a frequent occurrence during your investigations.

The results of these comparisons will then be used to make decisions regarding your health theory. Some suggestions are now made which may help you when making comparisons.

It may prove useful to employ some sort of rating system so that you can make meaningful comparisons which will then lead to you making balanced decisions.

You could choose a 5 star rating system, award marks out of 10 or assign a percentage.

Such systems can then be used to rank objects or activities.

For example, awarding articles a trustworthiness percentage will make it easy to rank the numerous articles which you have read on a particular topic.

By using some sort of rating system the process of decision making is also simplified as you merely select the highest rated option.

Motivation

One of the most important aspects of a robust health theory is that it is sustainable.

To help maintain the implementation of your health theory, it may also be useful to examine your motivation for doing so.

Some common motivating factors for following your healthy lifestyle in the long term include:
- body image
- fitness
- living longer
- medical issues
- our nearest and dearest

By clearly stating the factors that motivate you to design, construct and implement your health theory, you will have increased your chances of successfully maintaining your healthy lifestyle in the long term.

Maintaining motivation

Monitoring your progress can be a very powerful way of staying motivated.

It can also be very useful to set yourself goals.

To avoid disappointment and the potential for a subsequent decline in motivation, you should ensure that the goals which you set yourself are both realistic and achievable.

However, no matter how great your progress, it is inevitable that the initial rates of progress will eventually slow or indeed, stop.

It is therefore important to think about how you will maintain motivation when your goals are reached or when your progress slows or stops.

In the long term, a useful mantra might be:
- set a target
- reach it
- maintain it

Conducting trials

While designing and constructing your health theory it may prove useful to carry out your own trials to test various aspects of your health theory. For example, when trying a new exercise programme or a change in your diet.

When conducting any trial it is important that all other factors which could have an impact on the outcome of the trial remain unchanged.

This notion is commonly referred to by the Latin phrase **ceteris paribus**, which means "*all other things being equal*".

Remembering this *ceteris paribus* idea, you should aim to change only one aspect of your lifestyle per trial so that all other factors remain unchanged.

The appendix at the end of the book contains blank trial outlines so that you can keep track of your trials in a systematic manner.

Professional help

When designing and building your perfect home you would most likely employ the services of a wide variety of professionals.

Of course this book takes a DIY approach to the design and construction of your health theory, however, that doesn't mean you shouldn't consult various professionals along the way to get their expert guidance and advise.

Such specialists include:
- doctors
- pharmacists
- nutritionists
- personal trainers
- counsellors
- motivational specialists

Framework

Framework

In this part of the book the various factors which you might well consider when designing your health theory are set out and described.

Even if you do not feel that a factor is relevant to you it may still be useful to examine such a factor as you may discover something which you had not previously considered.

The section headings in this part are:
- Nutrition
- Exercise
- Hydration
- Smoking
- Alcohol
- Mental health & stress
- Sleep
- Common preventable diseases
- Regular medical checks
- Other considerations

Nutrition

Nutrition

Nutrition relates to the way you acquire all of the nutrients which your body needs to function, repair and grow.

Nutrition will be examined by considering each of the following topics in turn:
- Food constituents
- Basic dietary classes
- Food types
- Food prep & portioning
- Food allergies & intolerances

Note that in the next part of the book, where you design your own health theory, the focus of the nutrition section will be the sources of nutrients and how you can incorporate a wider variety of nutrient sources into your diet.

Food constituents
Carbohydrate: Starch

The first of the three main types of carbohydrate is starch.

Starch is a type of carbohydrate which is a white powder when dried and is primarily found in most cereals and potatoes.

The main function of starch in our diet is to provide energy.

Common names for starch which can appear on ingredient lists include:
- dextrin
- maltodextrin
- corn syrup

Food constituents
Carbohydrate: Sugar

The second main type of carbohydrate is sugar.

Sugar is a sweet tasting carbohydrate which is primarily derived from sugar cane and sugar beet.

Like starch, the main function of sugar in our diet is to provide energy.

Common names for sugar which can appear on ingredient lists include:
- glucose
- dextrose
- fructose
- galactose
- sucrose
- maltose
- lactose

Naturally occurring sugar alternatives include:
- sorbitol
- xylitol

Artificial sugar substitutes include:
- aspartame
- saccharin

Food constituents
Carbohydrate: Fibre

The third main type of carbohydrate is fibre *(US: fiber)*.

Fibre is a carbohydrate which is resistant to digestion by the body.

The main purpose of fibre in our diet is to aid the transit of food through the digestive system.

Common names for fibre which can appear on ingredient lists include:

- cellulose
- xanthan
- pectin
- lignin
- agar
- carrageen
- chitin

Food constituents
Fat

Fats are oily substances which can be found in both plant and animal based foods.

The two main functions of fat in our diet are to:
- provide energy
- store energy

Fats can be classified into two broad types:
- saturated fats
- unsaturated fats

Note that fat is an essential part our diet.

However, some types of fat have better health implications than others.

As a result, we will now examine each of the different types of fat.

Food constituents
Types of fat

Saturated fats are usually solid at room temperature.

Many health agencies advise people to lower their intake of saturated fats.

Unsaturated fats are usually liquid at room temperature and can be further classified as follows:
- mono-unsaturated fats
- poly-unsaturated fats
- trans-fats
- essential fatty acids

The health implications of each of the unsaturated fats are more varied.

For example, consumption of essential fatty acids is encouraged whereas many health agencies advise people to minimise their intake of trans-fats.

As a result, it may be advisable for you to carry out further research into the positive and negative effects of each of the different types of unsaturated fat.

Food constituents
Essential fatty acids

Essential fatty acids (EFAs) cannot be synthesised within your body and so they must be obtained from your diet.

There are two types of EFAs:
- omega-3 acids
- omega-6 acids

Other fatty acids, including omega-7 and omega-9, are not deemed essential as they can be produced within your body.

Common examples of EFAs include:
- **omega-3**
  ALA, EPA, DPA and DHA
- **omega-6**
  linoleic and arachidonic acid

Food constituents
Protein

Protein is an essential nutrient found in both plant and animal based foods.

The main functions of protein in our diet are to:
- aid growth of cells
- help in the repair of cells
- provide energy

Protein can be obtained from a wide variety of sources ranging from red meat and eggs to lentils and quinoa.

Protein consists of amino acids which we will now examine more closely.

Food constituents
Amino acids

There are nine amino acids which are classified as essential:

- histidine
- isoleucine
- leucine
- lysine
- methionine
- phenylalanine
- threonine
- tryptophan
- valine

As our body cannot synthesise these acids they must be obtained from our diet.

All essential amino acids are obtained directly from the protein in our diet.

It is worth noting that different protein sources contain different amounts of each essential amino acid.

As a result, obtaining protein from a wide variety of sources may be desirable.

Food constituents
Salt

Salt normally refers to sodium chloride, NaCl, and is an essential part of our diet.

The main functions of salt in our diet are to:
- aid nerve and muscle function
- regulate fluid balance within the body

Salt is essential to our survival, however, the WHO recommends that adults consume no more that 5 grams of salt per day.

There is a long established link between high salt consumption and high blood pressure.

Food constituents
Vitamins

A vitamin is a chemical compound which our body requires but cannot produce.

This means that sufficient quantities of each the following necessary vitamins must be obtained from our diet.
- Vitamin A
- Vitamins B_1, B_2, B_3, B_5, B_6, B_7, B_9 and B_{12}
- Vitamin C
- Vitamin D
- Vitamin E
- Vitamin K

It may be useful to research the various functions of each vitamin.

Vitamins can sometimes appear on ingredient lists under their scientific name, for example:
- Vitamin A : Retinol, retinal, beta-carotene
- Vitamin B_1 : Thiamin
- Vitamin B_2 : Riboflavin
- Vitamin B_3 : Niacin
- Vitamin B_7 : Biotin
- Vitamin B_9 : Folic acid, folate
- Vitamin C : Ascorbic acid

Food constituents
Minerals

Dietary minerals are chemical elements which are required by our body.

The main required elements include:
- calcium
- chlorine
- magnesium
- phosphorus
- potassium
- sodium
- sulphur

Other elements, known as trace elements, which are also required by our body, though in smaller quantities, include:
- bromine
- cobalt
- copper
- iron
- iodine
- manganese
- molybdenum
- selenium
- zinc

Again, it may be useful to research the various functions of each mineral.

Food constituents
Vitamin & mineral supplements

It is generally accepted by the medical community that a balanced diet should not ordinarily require the addition of vitamin and mineral supplements.

The only exceptions to this view are women who are in the first 3 months of pregnancy and women who are trying to conceive. Both of these groups are advised by the medical community to take **400 μg** (micrograms) of **folic acid** (vitamin B_9 or folate) every day.

Vitamins and minerals can occur in various foodstuffs in different forms and it is worth noting that these different forms of the same vitamin or mineral can be absorbed differently by the body.

For example, the iron in red meat is more readily absorbed than the iron in plants.

This means that identifying multiple sources of each vitamin and mineral may be advisable.

Basic dietary classes

When attempting to design a health theory and healthy lifestyle, there are essentially four broad choices for the type of diet that can be followed.

These four basic dietary classes are as follows:
- "Balanced" diet
- Vegetarian diet
- Pescetarian diet
- Vegan diet

We now examine each of these four classes in some detail.

Basic dietary classes
"Balanced" diet

The phrase "*as part of a balanced diet*" is one we hear almost every day.

But what exactly is a "balanced" diet?

Probably the most common "balanced" diet is the **Food Pyramid**.

Details vary between countries but the Food Pyramid can be summarised as follows:
- **no more than 2** servings per **week** of foods and drinks high in fat, sugar and/or salt
- **very small** servings of fats, spreads or oils
- **2** servings per **day** of meat, poultry, fish, shellfish, eggs, beans or nuts
- **3** servings per **day** of milk, cheese and/or yoghurt
- **3-5** servings per **day** of bread, rice, potatoes, pasta and/or cereals (wholegrain)
- **5-7** servings per **day** of fruit and vegetables

For the actual size of each serving you should consult your government's Department of Health webpage.

Basic dietary classes
Vegetarian diet

A vegetarian diet is essentially the same as the "balanced" diet minus the:
- meat
- poultry
- fish
- shellfish

As a result of not eating meat, poultry, fish or shellfish, all the nutrients which these foods provide will have to be replaced.

It is therefore important to identify vegetarian sources of the nutrients which are provided in the "balanced" diet by meat, poultry, fish and shellfish.

Basic dietary classes
Pescetarian diet

A pescetarian diet is essentially the same as the "balanced" diet minus the:
- meat
- poultry

Nutrients which are supplied by meat and poultry in the "balanced" diet will have to be acquired from other pescetarian sources.

It may be worth investigating the Japanese diet. The Japanese represent approximately 2% of the world's population and yet they consume almost 10% of the world's annual seafood production.

Basic dietary classes
Vegan diet

A vegan diet consists entirely of plant-based foods and contains no products derived from animals.

As with the vegetarian and pescetarian diets, it is important to identify alternative sources of the various nutrients which are provided by products derived from animals in the "balanced" diet.

Some essential nutrients which are not easily acquired when following a vegan diet include:
- heme-type iron
- biologically active vitamin B_{12}
- the essential fatty acids EPA and DHA

Food types
Organic produce

Products certified as organic must be produced in accordance with a list of standards which vary between countries.

Although these standards vary, in general the following are prohibited:
- artificial fertilisers
- chemical pesticides
- antibiotic use in animals
- growth hormone use in animals
- genetically modified (GM) ingredients
- artificial food additives
- irradiation of foodstuffs

Scientific research to establish any potential health benefits of consuming organic produce has thus far been inconclusive.

Food types
Unprocessed foods

Commonly referred to as natural or whole foods, unprocessed foods generally have either a single ingredient or else a very small number of simple ingredients and no artificial additives.

Using unprocessed foods as ingredients when cooking means that it is possible to have more control over both the quality and the quantity of the ingredients in each meal.

Using unprocessed foods when cooking also makes it easier to implement specific dietary changes, for example, reducing salt or saturated fat intake.

Food types
Processed foods

Any food item which is sold in a wrapper and contains more than one ingredient can be considered a processed food.

Normally the more ingredients in a food item, the higher the degree of processing.

It may be useful to read the list of ingredients on the wrapper of a food item and see if you recognise all of the ingredients.

Processed foods can contain high levels of:
- salt
- highly processed fats such as trans-fats or hydrogenated vegetable oil
- refined sugars such as corn syrup

It is worth noting that many products which are labelled *low-fat, low-calorie, low-sugar* or *diet*, can in fact be highly processed and may contain many processed ingredients and artificial food additives.

Food additives are substances which are added to foods for a specific purpose.

Common food additive categories include:
- preservatives
- stabilisers
- emulsifiers
- flavourings and flavour enhancers
- sweeteners
- thickeners
- artificial colours

Food additives are regulated in:
- Europe by the EU and each additive is identified by a unique E-number
- the US by the Food and Drug Administration (FDA)

It is worth noting that nearly all processed foods contain at least some food additives.

Food prep & portioning
Cooking methods

It may be useful to investigate the health implications of each of the following cooking methods:

- baking
- barbecuing
- deep frying
- grilling/broiling
- microwaving
- poaching
- pressure cooking
- raw food methods
- roasting
- shallow frying
- slow cooking
- steaming
- stir frying

Food prep & portioning
Portion size

The amount of food that we eat can be just as important as the type of food that we eat.

It is important to find out exactly what constitutes a portion of each type of food.

By using measuring cups and/or weighing scales it may be an interesting exercise to see how your estimate of a normal portion of a food compares with a recommended portion size for that food.

There are numerous potential long-term risks associated with consistently eating oversized portions.

These risks include:
- obesity
- heart disease
- type 2 diabetes

Food prep & portioning
Blood sugar & the glycemic index

The Glycemic Index (GI) rating of a food describes the speed at which that food raises blood sugar (and subsequently, insulin) levels.

GI ratings run from 0 to 100, where pure glucose has a GI of 100.

Insulin is produced by the pancreas and is needed by cells to absorb glucose.

The higher the GI of a food then the quicker the increase in blood sugar levels.

Quicker increases in blood sugar levels result in greater demands for insulin and so greater stresses are placed on the pancreas.

Prolonged stress on the pancreas can have a detrimental effect on pancreatic function, which can in turn lead to type 2 diabetes.

Food prep & portioning
Blood sugar & portion size

The more of a food we consume then the more our blood sugar level is elevated.

Therefore, it is important to not only consider the GI of a food, but also the quantity of that food which you consume.

It is desirable to maintain relatively stable blood sugar levels, as this avoids sharp spikes in insulin production and so avoids unnecessary stresses on the pancreas.

To avoid these spikes in insulin production it may be worth considering replacing large infrequent meals with smaller more frequent meals.

Food allergies & intolerances
Food allergies

A food allergy causes the immune system to react to an apparently harmless food.

Food allergies symptoms include breathing difficulties, stomach upsets and/or skin rashes.

A severe allergic reaction is called **anaphylaxis** and can be fatal.

People diagnosed with severe allergies normally carry adrenalin injections in case of anaphylaxis.

The most common food allergens include:
- nuts
- fish and shellfish
- eggs
- soya
- wheat
- milk

Careful reading of food labels and ingredients is very important not only for allergy sufferers but also for those who may be preparing food for allergy suffers.

Food allergies & intolerances
Food intolerances

A food intolerance causes a chemical reaction in the body to some food or drink.

The symptoms of mild to moderate food intolerances and allergies can be similar, but food intolerances do not cause anaphylaxis.

Symptoms of an allergy usually appear much more quickly than reactions due to a food intolerance.

The most common food intolerances include:
- dairy products
- wheat and gluten
- yeast
- eggs

Tests are available for a wide variety of food intolerances.

Further advise on such tests can be acquired from a doctor, nutritionist or pharmacist.

Food allergies & intolerances
Coeliac disease

Coeliac disease *(US: celiac disease)* is an autoimmune disease in which gluten causes the production of certain chemicals within the body which then trigger an adverse response from the immune system.

Coeliac disease can only be diagnosed by a doctor following a blood test and a biopsy (which is carried out using an endoscope).

At present, the only known treatment for coeliac disease is to follow a gluten-free diet.

It is still unclear if following a gluten-free diet has any health benefits for someone who does not suffer from coeliac disease.

Note that coeliac disease is not the same as wheat intolerance and/or yeast intolerance.

Exercise

Benefits of exercise

It is difficult to overstate the benefits of physical exercise.

The main benefits of exercise include:
- increased strength and fitness
- improved heart and lung function

Additional benefits of exercise include:
- better sleep quality
- improved mental health
- reduced stress levels
- increased self-confidence

The WHO recommends that adults take at least 150 minutes of exercise per week with muscle-strengthening activities undertaken at least twice per week.

Types of exercise

Exercise can be classified into the following three broad categories:
- cardiovascular/aerobic
- strength
- flexibility

Cardiovascular and aerobic exercise works the heart, circulatory system and the lungs.

Strength training usually involves targeting specific muscles or groups of muscles.

Flexibility training involves twisting and stretching.

Any good quality exercise programme should include all three types of exercise.

Getting more exercise

Exercise is a crucial part of any health theory and so ensuring that sufficient time is allocated to physical exercise will be vital.

To ensure that as much exercise as possible is incorporated into your health theory consider the following suggestions:
- choose physical activities which you find enjoyable
- consider team or group activities as you will be more likely to continue these activities than if you are on your own
- try to reduce the amount of time spent sitting down
- small but consistent changes will make a difference, for example, using the stairs on a daily basis instead of taking the lift
- set goals to work towards

Sedentary lifestyle

A sedentary lifestyle is characterised by a lack of regular physical activity and normally involves being seated for most of the day.

A sedentary lifestyle has been shown to increase the risk of many conditions including:
- high blood pressure
- cardiovascular disease
- depression
- obesity
- diabetes
- breast cancer
- colon cancer
- stroke

A sedentary lifestyle has also been linked to having a weaker immune system as well as having weaker bones.

Hydration

Water

Water accounts for between a half and two thirds of our body weight.

Water is the main constituent in bodily fluids, such as blood. Maintaining adequate levels of these fluids is vital as they facilitate many of the vital processes within the body.

Water is also a key component in the work of the kidneys which cleanse the body of waste.

Water is also crucial to the digestion of food and absorption of nutrients into the bloodstream.

Most health authorities recommend drinking approximately 2 litres or 4 pints of water per day, or enough to ensure that urine is light yellow or clear.

Coffee & tea

Common alternatives to water as a hydration source are coffee and tea.

Two important issues relating to coffee and tea consumption should be considered.

The first issue relates to the calorific values of coffee and tea.

When taken black, coffee and tea are both effectively calorie free. However, the addition of sugar, cream and/or syrups etc. can make these drinks a significant portion of your daily calorie intake. For example, compare the number of calories in a full-fat latte with syrup and whipped cream to the number of calories in a black Americano.

The second issue is that both coffee and tea contain the stimulant caffeine.

Stimulants such as caffeine elevate both heart rate and blood pressure and so it may be wise to consider the potential long-term effects of caffeine.

Soft drinks

Soft drinks *(US: sodas)* are another common source of hydration.

The main health concerns associated with soft drinks generally relate to their high sugar content.

Many of these drinks, particularly energy and sports drinks, also contain caffeine and/or other stimulants.

Although *diet* versions of many soft drinks are available, in these drinks the sugar is simply replaced by artificial sweeteners.

What is important to note however, is that *diet* and *regular* soft drinks are both highly acidic. As a result, it is worth being mindful of the detrimental impact which these drinks can have on your dental health.

Smoking

The statistics

Smoking has been the subject of much statistical research over the past half century or more.

The British Doctors Study followed over 40,000 British doctors from 1951 until 2001.

This study was one of the first to provide strong statistical evidence that smoking:
- increased the risk of heart-attack
- increased the risk of lung cancer
- decreased life expectancy
- was the main contributing factor in the deaths of 50% of smokers

Many other studies have provided evidence for the links between smoking and various other diseases. It may be useful to seek out and read the results of some of these studies.

The chemistry

Laboratory analyses have identified over 4000 different chemicals in tobacco smoke.

These chemicals include:
- ammonia
- arsenic
- benzene
- hydrogen cyanide
- polonium-210 (a radioactive substance)

Tobacco smoke also contains tar.

Tar is a viscous and sticky byproduct of burning tobacco and it is what causes the discolouration of a smoker's teeth and fingers, as well as causing lung damage.

The biology

Numerous studies over the years have found strong evidence that:

- smoking is harmful to almost every part of the human body
- smoking is the root cause of numerous diseases including many cancers
- smokers have lower recovery and survival rates after surgery
- smoking exacerbates the effects of other medical conditions

The main biological reason why smoking remains prevalent is that tobacco smoke contains the addictive chemical nicotine.

As with any addictive substance, giving up nicotine may be difficult and normally requires a committed and concerted effort.

The psychology

It is important to note that the addictive properties of nicotine are not the sole reason people continue to smoke.

As a result, it may be useful to examine the more subtle psychological, behavioural and social issues which contribute to a person's decision to continue smoking.

Many smokers associate having a cigarette with certain activities, for example, after eating or while drinking alcohol or coffee. These associations can make quitting smoking more difficult.

It is also vital to remember that people will continue to do things which they enjoy.

Therefore, as most smokers enjoy the experience and the immediate effects of smoking, it will be important to establish a compelling reason or reasons to stop smoking.

Alcohol

Overview

Alcohol consumption and the associated effects on our physical and mental health are both complex issues.

A significant amount of evidence exists which highlights the negative effects of excessive alcohol consumption on both our physical and mental health.

Excessive alcohol consumption also has negative social and economic effects.

It may also be worth noting that studies do exist which identify some positive health effects of moderate alcohol consumption.

The one key point of agreement amongst almost all health professionals when it comes to alcohol consumption can be described in a single word:

moderation

Alcohol & physical health

Excessive alcohol consumption is a significant risk factor in conditions such as:
- liver disease
- heart attack
- stroke
- high blood pressure

Alcohol consumption has also been linked to an increased risk of developing cancer along the digestive tract and in both the liver and the breast.

Excessive alcohol consumption can also complicate the treatment of other conditions.

Alcohol consumption during pregnancy is strongly discouraged due to the risk of developmental problems in the unborn child.

The most commonly reported positive physical effect of alcohol is an apparent link between moderate red wine consumption and lower rates of cardiovascular disease.

Alcohol & mental health

Alcohol has been linked to the development of mental health problems and it can compound existing mental health issues.

Alcohol and depression have a complex relationship and alcohol is known to be a factor in a significant proportion of suicides.

Excessive alcohol consumption can cause aggressive behaviour which can then give rise to a wide variety of negative outcomes.

Alcohol consumption affects our decision making ability and can lead to an increase in risk taking behaviour which can then result in:
- being involved in preventable accidents
- contracting preventable diseases

Commonly cited positive effects of alcohol consumption include aiding relaxation and reducing feelings of stress as well as enabling more enjoyable social interaction.

Mental health & stress

Mental health & stress

At first glance, this chapter may not seem relevant to you, however, it is worth noting that stress and mental health problems can both develop over time.

As with most health conditions, if these problems are recognised at an early stage, and appropriate measures taken, then the outcomes can be much improved.

It is therefore important to be aware of how to recognise the early symptoms of both stress and other issues which can adversely affect your mental health.

It will be much easier to recognise these symptoms if you know what they look like.

Stress

Stress is a very general term but it can be defined as:

A state of mental or emotional strain or tension which results from adverse or challenging circumstances.

Common sources of stress include:
- personal relationships
- medical issues
- work related issues
- financial issues
- the immediate environment (e.g. traffic)

Of course there can be many more sources of stress and so taking some time to identify the most common triggers of stress in your life, so that you can then try to avoid them, may be a beneficial exercise.

Recognising stress

It will be impossible to combat stress if you cannot identify when exactly you are experiencing stress.

It is also very important to remember that stress affects everyone differently.

Stress can manifest itself in a variety of different ways, common examples of which include:
- increased blood pressure
- sleeplessness
- headaches

As the symptoms of stress are both varied and numerous then it may be useful to search for common symptoms of stress and see which symptoms are most relevant to you.

Combatting stress

It is likely that different stressful situations will have to be addressed in different ways.

For example, it is likely that the stress experienced while commuting and the stress experienced in personal relationships will have to be addressed in completely different ways.

Therefore, it may be wise to build up a wide range of methods for combatting a whole spectrum of stressful situations.

Some methods worth considering include:
- exercise
- meditation
- relaxation
- talking about the situation
- practising good time-management
- mindfulness

Depression

Depression is a very broad term but can be described as follows:

A mental condition which can be characterised by feelings of despair and inadequacy, and is typically accompanied by low energy levels and a lack of interest in life.

The WHO estimate that approximately 350 million people (that is almost 5% of the world's population!) have suffered from depression over the past year.

As depression can range in severity from mild feelings of inadequacy to complete despair there are also a wide range of approaches to treating the condition.

Recognising depression

Recognising the symptoms of depression is very important as this should then prompt you to take steps to tackle the illness.

Depression can manifest itself in some or all of the following ways:
- persistent sadness
- poor self-confidence
- lack of interest in, or enjoyment of, daily life
- feelings of guilt, anxiety or worry
- thinking about harming yourself
- low-energy and fatigue
- sleeplessness

Note that there are numerous other ways in which depression can present itself and so you should conduct a search with the aim of compiling a more extensive list of symptoms.

If you are experiencing some or all of these symptoms, on a regular or prolonged basis, then you should **consult your doctor** as soon as possible.

Addressing depression

The effects of depression can vary widely and so there exists a wide variety of treatments for the condition, some of which do not involve medication.

In some cases of mild to moderate depression, symptoms may be alleviated through a combination of:
- eating healthily
- taking regular exercise
- speaking with a counsellor
- attending support group meetings

It is important to note here that these alternatives to medical treatment and medication are generally only useful in treating some cases of mild to moderate depression.

Again, if you have any concerns relating to depression, consult your doctor.

Socialising

We are naturally social animals.

As children we learn important life skills by interacting socially with others and as adults we can continue to learn through similar interactions.

Human contact and interaction can also be beneficial for our mood and mental wellbeing.

In particular, laughter has be shown to increase production of the hormone dopamine in the brain, which in turn results in feelings of happiness and pleasure.

Numerous studies have also found evidence to suggest that living alone, particularly over a number of years, can be detrimental to both our physical and mental health.

Continued education

Continued education can involve learning more about any subject which interests you and does not necessarily involve acquiring new work-related skills or knowledge.

In fact, *"knowledge for knowledge's sake"* is a long held mantra in academic circles.

Learning is a challenging activity which requires concentrated thought and so it promotes mental sharpness and agility.

By setting and achieving goals, the process of learning can also provide a sense of purpose and give a feeling of fulfilment.

Continued education can also be a source of improved self-esteem and self-confidence.

Religion & spirituality

Religion and spirituality can be of vital importance to some people while being totally irrelevant to others.

When dealing with challenging circumstances or events some people take solace and comfort in religion and spirituality while others find solace and comfort elsewhere.

If you consider yourself religious or spiritual then perhaps examine how these beliefs can help you deal with stress as well as other health and mental health related issues.

The role of religion and spirituality in health related issues has been studied extensively and you may find it worthwhile to seek out the findings of some of these studies.

If you are not religious or spiritual then clearly religion and spirituality will not play any part in your health theory.

Attitude & outlook

It may be worth considering the role that your attitude and outlook on life plays in your physical and mental health.

Would you consider yourself to be:
- **optimistic**
  do you normally see the good in situations and have a positive outlook on life?
- **pessimistic**
  do you normally see the bad in situations and have a negative outlook on life?
- **realistic**
  do you normally deal with situations in a detached manner and have neither a positive nor a negative outlook on life?

Some studies have found evidence to suggest that a positive attitude benefits both your physical and mental health. Perhaps try to find some of these studies and examine the details.

Sleep

Sleep

Sleep is one of the most important and fundamental activities which we undertake on a daily basis.

Even if you do not have any sleep related issues at present, it is possible that you may experience sleep problems in the future.

Sleep problems can occur because of stress, during challenging circumstances or as a result of other health problems.

This section aims to increase your awareness of both the importance of sleep and the negative effects which sleep problems can have on your health.

The importance of sleep

The mechanics of what actually happens when we sleep are not yet fully understood.

However, there is no question about the importance of sleep.

It is widely accepted that the main functions of sleep are to facilitate the:
- regeneration of cells
- repair of damaged cells
- consolidation of information within the brain

Various studies have highlighted the vital role played by sleep in both memory function and the learning process.

Lack of sleep

Studies have linked sleep problems to higher instances of various conditions, including heart disease, stroke and even obesity.

Sleep problems can also have detrimental effects on your:
- memory function
- alertness
- mental health
- physical performance
- mood
- decision making ability

As a lack of sleep can impair your alertness and decision making, there is an increased risk of being involved in accidents. This is particularly true of road traffic accidents.

Some studies have found evidence to suggest that it is not possible to "catch-up" on sleep.

Sleeplessness

Sleeplessness, or insomnia, makes it difficult for a person to fall asleep or to remain asleep.

Some of the many possible causes of sleeplessness include:
- anxiety
- stress
- depression
- irregular working hours or shift work
- poor sleep environment
- certain medical conditions or medications
- stimulants such as caffeine

Although possible remedies usually depend on the specific cause, some general methods to combat sleeplessness include:
- learning relaxation methods
- taking physical exercise
- limiting caffeine/stimulant intake
- ensuring your bedroom is quiet and dark

Your bedroom

Most people sleep between 6 and 8 hours per day.

This means that you spend between 25% and 33% of your life in bed.

To ensure that you get good quality sleep then the main factors to consider in your bedroom are your:
• mattress
• pillow
• blinds and curtains

Considering the large proportion of your time that is spent in bed then it may be worthwhile investing some time and money when selecting your mattress and pillow.

It is also worth ensuring that your bedroom is dark. To achieve this it may be useful to consider blackout blinds or heavy dark-coloured curtains.

You should also try to ensure that your bedroom is a quiet as possible so that your sleep is not interrupted.

Many sleep experts also advise against having any electronic devices with screens in your bedroom.

Common preventable diseases

Common preventable diseases

The key point of this section can be summed up in just five words:

Prevention is better than cure

We will examine lifestyle risk factors and preventative steps which can be taken in relation to the following five common diseases:
- heart disease
- type 2 diabetes
- skin cancer
- lung cancer
- cirrhosis of the liver

Most cases of these diseases are preventable.

Furthermore, these five diseases are among the most common causes of death in the developed world today.

You should also inform yourself about other preventable diseases and their risk factors.

Heart disease

Lifestyle related risk factors for developing heart disease include:
- having high blood pressure
- having high cholesterol
- smoking
- having diabetes
- being overweight or obese

Simple lifestyle changes which can help prevent heart disease include:
- following a low-fat healthy diet
- getting regular aerobic exercise
- stopping smoking
- losing weight

It is worth noting that heart disease and stroke have very similar lifestyle risk factors and preventative methods.

Type 2 diabetes

Lifestyle related risk factors for developing type 2 diabetes include:
- being overweight or obese
- not getting regular physical exercise
- having high blood sugar levels

Simple lifestyle changes which can help prevent type 2 diabetes include:
- losing weight
- getting regular aerobic exercise
- following a (low-GI) healthy diet

Diabetes is not only a serious condition itself, but it can also cause complications in the treatment of many other medical conditions.

Skin cancer

Lifestyle related risk factors for developing skin cancer include:
- regular exposure to the sun
- regular use of tanning-salons/sun-beds

Note that people with fair skin and blond or red hair are most at risk of developing skin cancer.

Simple lifestyle changes which can help prevent skin cancer include:
- regularly applying suncream
- staying out of direct sunlight between noon and 3pm
- wearing clothing to cover sensitive skin
- covering moles completely
- avoid using tanning-salons/sun-beds

You should consult your doctor as soon as possible if you notice any changes in the size, colour or texture of a mole.

Lung cancer

Lifestyle related risk factors for developing lung cancer include:
- smoking
- passive smoking

Simple lifestyle changes which can help prevent lung cancer include:
- stopping smoking
- avoiding passive smoking

Environmental risk factors for developing lung cancer include exposure to:
- asbestos
- radon gas

Testing kits for the level of radon gas in your home are widely available.

Cirrhosis of the liver

Lifestyle related risk factors for developing cirrhosis of the liver include:
- excessive alcohol consumption
- being overweight or obese
- having diabetes

Simple lifestyle changes which can help prevent cirrhosis of the liver include:
- reducing alcohol consumption
- losing weight
- following a healthy diet

Another significant risk factor for cirrhosis of the liver is suffering from hepatitis B or C.

Search for information relating to the different types of hepatitis and how each type can be contracted and prevented.

Regular medical checks

Regular medical checks

The importance of this section can be summed up by the old adage:

A stitch in time saves nine

It is widely accepted in the medical community that, in general, the earlier a disease is diagnosed or detected then the better the prognosis or likely outcome.

Of course it is not feasible to have regular checks for a whole array of diseases and conditions.

However, it may be advisable, particularly as we get older, to regularly undergo some or all of the following common and relatively inexpensive checks.

Your doctor is the best person to advise you as to which tests are most relevant to you.

Regular medical checks

Weight & Body Mass Index

Noticing gradual changes in your own weight can be difficult and as a result changes in your weight can easily go unchecked.

To address this issue it may be a good idea to weigh yourself regularly (perhaps once a month) and to keep a record.

The easiest way to check for obesity is to find out your Body Mass Index (BMI) using an online BMI calculator.

Blood pressure & pulse

These simple tests, when carried out by a medical professional, can detect warning signs of other potentially serious conditions.

Examples include:
- High blood pressure can point to an increased risk of heart disease.
- An irregular pulse can signal an increased risk of stroke or heart attack.

Regular medical checks

Cholesterol

Cholesterol is a fat-like substance essential for our bodies to function. There are various types of cholesterol including LDL and HDL.

There are no symptoms associated with having high cholesterol levels.

Your cholesterol level can only be found via a blood test administered by your doctor who will then advise you on the results.

Anaemia

Anaemia *(US: anemia)* is a condition caused by a lack of red blood cells or haemoglobin.

The main symptoms of anaemia are persistent tiredness, feeling faint and lacking in energy.

Common causes of anaemia include iron deficiency and vitamin B_{12} deficiency.

Anaemia can be diagnosed by your doctor following a blood test.

Regular medical checks

Type 2 diabetes

Type 2 diabetes and the related risk factors have already been discussed.

Symptoms of diabetes include:
- commonly being thirsty
- increased urination

Diabetes can be diagnosed by your doctor using a simple blood test.

Moles

Moles are growths on the skin consisting of groups of pigment cells called melanocytes.

Moles should be checked regularly and you should notify your doctor immediately of any changes in the colour, size or texture of a mole, or if a mole becomes itchy or starts to bleed.

Such changes can be the first signs of melanoma, a particularly serious form of skin cancer, which is diagnosed following a biopsy of the mole.

Regular medical checks

Bowel cancer

Bowel cancer refers to a cancerous growth found in the colon, rectum or large intestine.

Common symptoms of bowel cancer include:
- blood in the stool
- changes in bowel movement

Bowel cancer is usually diagnosed after a colonoscopy which follows a preliminary rectal exam by your doctor and a subsequent stool sample analysis.

Osteoporosis

Osteoporosis means *porous bones* and causes bones to weaken and become fragile.

Common symptoms of osteoporosis include:
- a bone fracture caused by a minor trauma
- persistent back pain
- loss of height or developing a stoop

Numerous tests for osteoporosis exist and your doctor will advise you on these tests.

Regular medical checks

Eye checks

Opticians generally recommend having an eye exam at least once every two years.

In addition to a standard sight-test, your optician should perform a glaucoma test as well as other medical checks of your eyes.

If your optician observes any evidence of other medical issues then they will advise you about seeking further medical attention.

Dental checks

Dentists generally recommend having a dental check at least once a year.

In addition to a standard dental check, your dentist will also assess your general oral health, noting that symptoms of other health issues can be detected during an oral exam.

If your dentist observes any evidence of other medical issues then they will advise you about seeking further medical attention.

Regular medical checks
Female

Breast cancer

Breast cancer is the most commonly diagnosed cancer in women.

The two most common checks are:
- self-examination for lumps or tenderness
- mammogram i.e. an X-ray of the breast

Search for more information on both checks.

Men can develop breast cancer but it is rare.

Cervical cancer

The most common and reliable way of checking for cervical cancer is to regularly visit your doctor for a Pap smear test.

Search for more information on warning signs.

It is also advisable to search for more information about HPV vaccination and cervical cancer.

Regular medical checks
Male

Prostate cancer

Prostate cancer is the most commonly diagnosed cancer in men.

The most common and reliable check for prostate cancer is to regularly visit your doctor for a blood test to check PSA levels.

Search for more information on symptoms related to prostate cancer.

Testicular cancer

Testicular cancer is particularly responsive to treatment and this fact further highlights the importance of early detection.

The most common check for testicular cancer involves self-examination for lumps or tenderness.

Search for more information on symptoms and self-examination.

Other considerations

Other considerations

While researching your health theory, you may wish to consider issues relating to:

- morals
- ethics
- ideals and principles

Note that it may be difficult to measure the direct effects of such issues on your health.

Even so, you may feel that your overall health theory will benefit by considering such issues.

Some of these moral or ethical issues include:

- tackling waste
- the sourcing of products
- animal welfare

Waste

A large portion of our waste is preventable.

As well as this, another large portion of what we waste has the potential to be used again.

A current campaign to tackle waste addresses these two issues in just 3 words:
- **reduce**
- **reuse**
- **recycle**

It may be worth trying to incorporate the 3 prongs of this campaign into your daily life.

Note that some of the most commonly wasted resources include:
- food
- energy e.g. electricity and heat
- water

Responsible sourcing

Equitable sourcing

The main focus of equitable sourcing is to ensure that no person involved in producing the product has been exploited in any way.

Various initiatives exist which ensure fair pay and good working conditions for production workers, particularly in the developing world.

Sustainable sourcing

The main focus of sustainable sourcing is to ensure that no natural resource used to produce the product has been overexploited.

Common examples of resources for which initiatives exist to safeguard them against overexploitation include various species of fish as well as trees.

Responsible sourcing

Local sourcing

When determining your views on local sourcing, it may be worth considering the issue from an:
- economic perspective
- ecological perspective

Economically speaking, perhaps consider the effect that local sourcing has on:
- producers in your locality
- your local economy

Ecologically speaking, perhaps consider the effect that local sourcing has on the:
- carbon footprint of a product
- freshness of a food product

Animal welfare

Animal welfare is a wide and varied issue and may be incorporated into your health theory.

Some animal welfare issues relating to your food which may be worth considering include:
- ethical farming practices
- humane transportation methods
- humane slaughter methods

Other issues relating to animal welfare which may also be worth considering include:
- eating animal products
- wearing products derived from animals

Notes

My health theory

My health theory

This is the most important part of *my **health** theory.*

The section headings in this part mirror those in the previous Framework section of the book.

This part of the book contains mostly white space and so provides you with a place to write down your own personal health theory using the principles, tools and framework outlined in the previous sections of the book.

Before you begin to write your health theory it may be useful to examine your motivation for researching, designing and implementing your health theory.

My motivation

Reasons to research and design my health theory and then to implement and maintain a healthy lifestyle:

Maintaining motivation

Inspirational people:

Inspirational quotes:

Nutrition

Carbohydrate: Starch

Interesting information:

Healthy sources of starch:

How starch fits into my healthy lifestyle:

Carbohydrate: Sugar

Interesting information:

Healthy sources of sugar:

How sugar fits into my healthy lifestyle:

Carbohydrate: Fibre

Interesting information:

Healthy sources of fibre:

How fibre fits into my healthy lifestyle:

Fat: Saturated

Interesting information:

Healthy sources of saturated fat:

How saturated fat fits into my healthy lifestyle:

Fat: Unsaturated

Interesting information:

Healthy sources of unsaturated fat:

How unsaturated fat fits into my healthy lifestyle:

Fat: Essential fatty acids

Interesting information:

Healthy sources of EFAs:

How EFAs fit into my healthy lifestyle:

Protein

Interesting information:

Healthy sources of protein:

How protein fits into my healthy lifestyle:

Salt

Interesting information:

Healthy sources of salt:

Hidden sources of salt:

Alternatives to salt:

How salt fits into my healthy lifestyle:

Vitamins

List as many commonly available foods from which you can acquire each of the following vitamins:

Vitamin A :

Vitamin B_1 :

Vitamin B_2 :

Vitamin B_3 :

Vitamin B_5 :

Vitamin B_6 :

Vitamin B_7 :

Vitamin B_9 :

Vitamin B_{12} :

Vitamin C :

Vitamin D :

Vitamin E :

Vitamin K :

Minerals

List foods from which you can acquire each mineral:

Calcium :

Chlorine :

Magnesium :

Phosphorus :

Potassium :

Sodium :

Sulphur :

List foods containing each of the following trace elements:

Bromine :
Cobalt :
Copper :
Iron :
Iodine :
Manganese :
Molybdenum :
Selenium :
Zinc :

"Balanced" diet

Interesting information:

Positives:

Negatives:

How the "balanced" diet and Food Pyramid fit into my healthy lifestyle:

Vegetarian diet

Interesting information:

Positives:

Negatives:

How the vegetarian diet fits into my healthy lifestyle:

Pescetarian diet

Interesting information:

Positives:

Negatives:

How the pescetarian diet fits into my healthy lifestyle:

Vegan diet

Interesting information:

Positives:

Negatives:

How the vegan diet fits into my healthy lifestyle:

Organic produce

Interesting information:

Positives:

Negatives:

How organic produce fits into my healthy lifestyle:

Unprocessed foods

Interesting information:

Positives:

Negatives:

How unprocessed foods fit into my healthy lifestyle:

Processed foods

Interesting information:

Positives:

Negatives:

How processed foods fit into my healthy lifestyle:

Food Additives

Interesting information:

Positives:

Negatives:

How food additives fit into my healthy lifestyle:

Cooking methods

For each of the listed methods consider whether you should use this method more or less frequently in your healthier lifestyle:

- baking

- barbecuing

- deep frying

- grilling/broiling

- microwaving

- poaching

- pressure cooking

- raw food methods

- roasting

- shallow frying

- slow cooking

- steaming

- stir frying

Portion size

Recommended portion size of foods you regularly eat:

Tips to control portion size:

How portion sizing fits into my healthy lifestyle:

Blood sugar

Interesting information:

High GI foods:

Low GI foods:

How the glycemic index fits into my healthy lifestyle:

Food allergies & intolerances

Interesting information:

Information regarding food allergy and intolerance testing:

How food allergies and intolerances fit into my healthy lifestyle:

Exercise

Current amount of exercise

It may be useful to estimate how much exercise you take during an average week.

Day	Type	Duration
Monday		
Tuesday		
Wednesday		
Thursday		
Friday		
Saturday		
Sunday		
Total		

Getting more exercise

Physical activities which I enjoy:

Physical activities which I'd like to try:

Helpful tips to increase the amount of exercise I get:

Amount of sedentary activity

It may be useful to estimate how much time during an average day that you spend on the following sedentary activities.

Type	Duration
Watching TV	
Using a computer	
Playing computer games	
Driving	
Other seated activities	
Total	

Reducing sedentary time

Sedentary activities which I can reduce:

I can replace sedentary activities with:

Helpful tips to decrease the amount of my sedentary activities:

Hydration

My hydration habits

I should drink **more** of these beverages:

I should drink **less** of these beverages:

My hydration habits

Find out the pH level of the drinks you most commonly consume:

Note: Acids have a pH of between 0 (strong) and 6.9 (weak)

Helpful tips to increase overall hydration:

Smoking

Smoking facts

Compile a list chemicals which are contained in tobacco smoke:

Find an image on the internet of a lung taken from a smoker. Describe the image:

If you need further convincing of the harmful effects of smoking, exhale some tobacco smoke through a piece of spare white cloth. Describe the effect:

Quitting smoking

Should I quit smoking?

If you answered **YES**:

List your reasons to quit smoking:

Helpful tips which may help you quit smoking:

If you answered **NO**:

List your reasons for continuing to smoke. Ask yourself if each reason is valid:

Alcohol

Current alcohol intake

It may be a useful exercise to estimate your daily alcohol intake over the course of an average week.

Day	Type	Amount
Monday		
Tuesday		
Wednesday		
Thursday		
Friday		
Saturday		
Sunday		
Total		

Search for weekly guidelines on alcohol consumption and see how your consumption compares:

Reducing alcohol intake

List times when you could drink less alcohol:

List ways you could try to reduce your alcohol intake:

List possible alternatives to alcoholic beverages:

Mental health & stress

Stress

List the most common sources of your stress:

List the symptoms you most commonly experience when you feel stressed:

List possible methods to combat your stress:

Depression

Common symptoms of depression:

Ways to address mild depression:

If you feel that you are experiencing depression then you should consult your doctor.

Socialising

List the social events which you most enjoy:

List ways in which you could improve your social life:

Loneliness can be particularly acute amongst older people. Are there any older people that you could contact more frequently?

Continued education

Subjects which you find interesting:

Skills that you would like to learn or improve:

Resources that you can use to continue your education:

Religion & spirituality

Religion and/or spirituality help me deal with issues such as:

Interesting research results about the relationship between religion and/or spirituality and health:

Attitude & outlook

Consider each of the following:

Being an optimist:
- Pros:
- Cons:

Being a pessimist:
- Pros:
- Cons:

Being a realist:
- Pros:
- Cons

Interesting research results about the relationship between attitude/outlook and health:

Sleep

Sleep

It may be a useful exercise to note the duration and the quality of your sleep over an average week.

Day	Amount of sleep	Quality of sleep
Monday		
Tuesday		
Wednesday		
Thursday		
Friday		
Saturday		
Sunday		

Methods to combat sleeplessness:

Your bedroom

Ways to make my bedroom darker:

Ways to make my bedroom quieter:

Devices with screens I can remove from my bedroom:

What makes a good quality pillow?

What makes a good quality mattress?

Common preventable diseases

Common preventable diseases

Heart disease

Relevant risk factors:

Preventative measures:

Type 2 diabetes

Relevant risk factors:

Preventative measures:

Common preventable diseases

Skin cancer

Relevant risk factors:

Preventative measures:

Lung cancer

Relevant risk factors:

Preventative measures:

Cirrhosis of the liver

Relevant risk factors:

Preventative measures:

Regular
medical
checks

Regular medical checks

You can carry out these regular checks yourself:

Weight:
Weigh yourself and calculate your Body Mass Index (BMI) using an online BMI calculator

Date	Weight	BMI

Regular medical checks

Search for information on how to conduct self-examinations in each of the following cases.

Moles:

Female: **Breast exam**

Male: **Testicular exam**

Regular medical checks

Consider visiting your doctor for the following checks.

Cholesterol				
Date				
Time				

Anaemia				
Date				
Time				

Type 2 diabetes				
Date				
Time				

Cervical cancer				
Date				
Time				

Prostate cancer				
Date				
Time				

Regular medical checks

Consider visiting your optician for a regular check.

Eye examination				
Date				
Time				

Consider visiting your dentist for a regular check.

Dental examination				
Date				
Time				

Other considerations

Waste

Ways you can **REDUCE** your waste:

Ways you can **REUSE** more of your waste:

Ways you can **RECYCLE** more of your waste:

Responsible sourcing

Products which I will try to source **equitably**:

Products which I will try to source **sustainably**:

Animal welfare

Products I consume where animal welfare is an issue:

How animal welfare issues fit into my healthy lifestyle:

Appendix

Conducting trials

Remember, ceteris paribus! Change only one thing at a time and leave everything else unchanged.

The **ONE** change I'm testing:

Trial length:

Question	Answer
Did I notice any differences?	
Describe any differences	
Did the trial require a lot of time/effort?	
Did the trial cost me more money?	
Overall result	

Conducting trials

Remember, ceteris paribus! Change only one thing at a time and leave everything else unchanged.

The **ONE** change I'm testing:

Trial length:

Question	Answer
Did I notice any differences?	
Describe any differences	
Did the trial require a lot of time/effort?	
Did the trial cost me more money?	
Overall result	

Conducting trials

Remember, ceteris paribus! Change only one thing at a time and leave everything else unchanged.

The **ONE** change I'm testing:

Trial length:

Question	Answer
Did I notice any differences?	
Describe any differences	
Did the trial require a lot of time/effort?	
Did the trial cost me more money?	
Overall result	

Conducting trials

Remember, ceteris paribus! Change only one thing at a time and leave everything else unchanged.

The **ONE** change I'm testing:

Trial length:

Question	Answer
Did I notice any differences?	
Describe any differences	
Did the trial require a lot of time/effort?	
Did the trial cost me more money?	
Overall result	

Conducting trials

Remember, ceteris paribus! Change only one thing at a time and leave everything else unchanged.

The **ONE** change I'm testing:

Trial length:

Question	Answer
Did I notice any differences?	
Describe any differences	
Did the trial require a lot of time/effort?	
Did the trial cost me more money?	
Overall result	

Conducting trials

Remember, ceteris paribus! Change only one thing at a time and leave everything else unchanged.

The **ONE** change I'm testing:

Trial length:

Question	Answer
Did I notice any differences?	
Describe any differences	
Did the trial require a lot of time/effort?	
Did the trial cost me more money?	
Overall result	

Notes

Notes

Notes